I, VAGINA

An Insider's View of Sex & Orgasm

Ruby G.Ash

Dedicated To Lovers Everywhere

Relax, take your time, there's no rush.
Look. Explore. Touch. Smell. Taste.
The art of sex is in the detail. Get the small
stuff right and the rest will come naturally.
And often!

CONTENTS

INTRODUCTION

HELLO AND WELCOME to my moist little world, please allow me to introduce myself. My Owner calls me Ruby and seeing as her last name is Ash I guess that must make me Ruby Ash.

I assume at some point she thought it might be frightfully clever and amusing if she threw in the extra 'G'. Yeah, funny!

Don't tell her but I think Ruby is quite a cute little name, don't you? It has to be better than most of the names I've heard for a device like me, I rather like it.

To be frank, it sums me up quite well as I do tend to get a little 'flushed' when things start to hot up.

I won't tell you my Owner's first name to protect the innocent, but I'll try to give you a very basic picture. She's tall – a tad over six foot in her killer heels – slim and long-limbed.

She's got what I suppose you'd call a boyish figure: slim-hipped, gap between the thighs, perky little tits, that sort of thing. Not skinny like all the anorexic models you see, but not curvy either. How she keeps her figure I do not know because she eats like she knows there's a famine coming tomorrow.

All this is topped off by quite a striking and unruly mass of curly red hair. I'm sure you get the picture. I suppose you would call her girlishly pretty in a pale-skinned, freckly, Nicole-Kidman-with-attitude sort of way.

Age? Don't ask! She's old enough to know what she wants and young enough to get it. She can be a bit fiery and has very little patience for knob-heads, idiots and douche-bags.

Basically, she's your typical snarky redhead. As am I. I am her vagina.

This little book is all about me. It's about how I, and all the other bits in and around me, work. The whole sexual enchilada, as it were. (OK, unfortunate term, but it fits.)

It's also about how you and I are going to have to work together if we're both going to get what we want. More of that later.

This is not going to be a detailed technical manual of female anatomy so I am going to assume you know what a girl's sexy bits look like. If you don't, go ahead and Google it now, I'll wait...

Well that took longer than expected, you weren't self-loving while you studied, were you, you naughty boy? No? Okay, so I'll assume the real reason was that you were studying the subject carefully and taking notes. Good.

Then you will have noticed one major detail: every Ruby is unique, we all look different and we're all beautiful. We all smell differently and we all work differently too, though I doubt even the Great Gods of Google have the power to get those little points across.

The Vulva

So now you're an expert on the female sexual organs, you'll know that it's not just about the vagina, we have various other bits as well, like the clitoris, the labia, the mons and the perineum, all of which do a different job and come under the collective term of vulva.

Vulva? Who the hell was it that decided 'vulva' would be the best word to describe this thing we girls hold between our legs? A vulva is not something sexy and beautiful, a Vulva is a sad old Swedish car - safe, slow and boring.

Fuck that, that is so not me. I like to think of myself as something a bit more exciting than that, something that will fire the imagination and stir the blood. Let's dump the Vulva right now and find another word to describe a thing of beauty such as me.

And so, ladies and gentlemen (drum-roll)... introducing (still with the drum-roll)... the Furrara!

A sensuously-sleek thoroughbred in racing red. Exciting, temperamental and raring to go. From here on in we're going to fire up our Furrara and launch her, wheels spinning, down the road, leaving that sad old Vulva forever choking in our dust.

Go forth and spread this new word, sisters. Embrace it, own it, show it off wherever you can. Be proud of your shiny new Furrara.

But I digress.

Warning, bad language alert!

Here is a warning for those of a sensitive nature: You will have noticed that I don't pussy-foot around with words when I want to get my point across. To put it bluntly, I have a bit of a dirty mouth.

If you're offended by the 'F-word' or the 'C-word' you really shouldn't be reading a book about vaginas. Go away and do some knitting or something.

And while we're talking of the 'C-word', believe it or not my first thought for the title of this book was, I Am A Cunt. What? Nothing wrong with that, it's short, to the point and factually correct: everything a best-selling non-fiction title should be. I thought it was perfect.

Unfortunately, my Owner overruled me as she couldn't quite see retailers like Waterstones or WHSmith (huge UK booksellers) being too keen to give the book much prominence in their window displays. I suppose she had a point.

Anyway, I thought I'd write this book - with my Owner's help, obviously, I'm not that clever - purely for selfish reasons. Because I've had it up to here (use your imagination) with all the fumbling, inept, and downright abysmal treatment I've had to endure over the years since she became sexually active. Why she puts up with it, I do not know.

You guys really do need to learn how we vaginas

work, that way you can give me the right attention once you get your hands into her panties. I know some of you may have been here before but, let's face it, you haven't been doing too well up to now, have you?

How it all began

When it comes to sex and how to treat an Owner there's no mystery, you just need to understand she doesn't work in the same way as you. Basically, men want sex, women want love.

The art of pleasuring a woman does not come naturally to men. In fact, most men only open up and get in touch with their feelings after they've had sex. Unfortunately, a woman needs him to do it the other way round. She needs the touchy-feely thing first, before she's ready to let him in. This is just a legacy of our evolutionary past.

Since the dawn of time you guys have been hunters and lunch-providers, ever alert to see off the enemy, and always on the lookout for danger. You're genetically programmed to increase your 'tribe' by being ready for any chance encounter with a female.

But having sex makes you vulnerable to attack, you need to impregnate her quickly by getting to your climax as soon as you can, just in case a sabre-tooth tiger comes along and makes a meal out of you, or another male with a bigger club than yours happens by to hit you over the head and steal your prize.

Guys, I've got some seriously good news for you: unless you happen to be sitting in your undiscovered village deep in the Peruzillonian jungle, reading this book on a stone tablet, neither of these scenarios is ever likely to happen. So chill.

However, she's different, she's a nest-builder, a gatherer, programmed to nurture her brood, to keep them around her and protect them from harm, to always know where they are and be aware of their feelings and wants. She needs time and understanding - affection, touch, and gentle persuasion - before she lets you into her most secret places.

If you do her the honor of respecting that fact you will go far along the path of enlightenment and understanding. She will reveal to you her deepest feelings and desires. Then she will fuck you to a standstill!

So if you're a guy reading this, just sit back, relax and let my words soak in as you gradually build up your knowledge about me and improve your technique. Try to control your usual headlong rush to get to the juicy bit at the end. The middle bit is important, it is here where you will find the enlightenment you're looking for.

Just like reading, sex is all about starting at the introduction and opening chapters, sticking with it through the middle section and not stopping until you get to the climax and acknowledgements at the end. Can you see where I'm going with this? Good boy! If you can do this it will make me a very happy Ruby indeed.

If you're a girl reading this, you have a Ruby of your own. It will look, feel, react and smell completely differently to me. It's yours, it's a unique and beautiful thing. Explore it yourself, get to know all its secret little places, if you don't know what it does and how it works how can you expect your partner to?

But please, for your own sake, once you've read this book just make sure you give it to your man, then send him away and tell him not to come back until he's read it too. Better still, buy him his own copy, my Owner has to eat, you know!

Chapter 1

THIS IS ME

DUE TO YOUR EARLIER extensive research - either practical hands-on or theoretical via Google or wank mags - you will have discovered we Rubies are all different.

Some are neat and petite, others are happy and flappy; some are fresh and fragrant, others are down and dirty; some are smooth and shaved, others are richly forested; some clits take a bit of finding, others need no map or compass; some may need a bit of lube, others may need mopping up; some may be painfully tight, others may be like throwing a banana up Main Street.

The point is, it doesn't fucking matter what we look

like, we all just want the same thing: a bit of proper attention.

And please, get over the size thing, we'll adapt, we're good at that. It's not about you and whether your 'ego' is man enough, it's about us and whether you know what you're doing. Treat us right and we really don't give a shit how big your 'ego' is.

As this book is all about me, I suppose I'd better tell you a bit about myself, put a face to the name, so to speak.

I'm fairly neat and tidy to look at but my inner lips aren't shy, they like to hang out there a bit and strut their stuff, looking for a bit of action.

As I said earlier, I'm a redhead (a sort of gingery-blonde to be precise). I have a fine silky thatch up on my mound and I'm neatly trimmed around the business end. She likes me nicely covered everywhere and is not into the shaved look. I like this, it keeps me warm at night!

It also provides me with the proper place nature gave me to nurture my musky smells. You'll like that once you get down there. You do go down there, don't you? If you don't like going 'down there' you'd better fucking start liking it, and quick, because until you do you'll forever be a four-out-of-ten man when she puts those notches in the bedpost.

Being a redhead, her skin is quite pale so my lips and inner bits tend to be prominently pink. Once you've done your bit and warmed her up, my lips will tend to redden further and the outer ones will plump up. As well as this, my clit will have come nicely out to play.

I am also a bit of a gusher, by the time you get your hand in her panties they'll be wet - and I don't mean damp.

As you can see, I'm not the kind of Ruby that holds back, you'll definitely know when I'm ready!

What do I smell like? Gorgeously fucking sexy! Well what did you expect me to say, Sweat, stale piss and two-day-old cod?

How do you go about describing a smell anyway? I suppose, like any recipe, you start off with your list of basic ingredients and then you carefully blend them all together to produce your mouth-watering masterpiece.

So here goes: First we take a freshly-showered

armpit, then we leave it for four or five hours into the day so it gets all warm and musky. Then we add a dash of truffle oil, a dribble of champagne, a cherry and a couple of juicy raisins. Finally we add to this a bit of seaweed, an olive and a small quantity of finest Beluga caviar.

Cover with something silky and lacy, marinade for an hour or two, and that's me: I smell kinda earthy, winey, fruity, beachy and fishy.

Like I said, Gorgeously fucking sexy! Some guys will like this, some guys won't. Do I give a shit? Take me as I am or take a hike.

My Ruby sisters will all look and smell differently to me. If you're a clean freak you'll maybe want to go for a shaven haven belonging to an owner who never goes anywhere without her wet-wipes. If you like 'em down and dirty I'm sure you can find an owner who dribbles in her panties and wipes herself from back to front. Hey, I'm just saying!

You might like your Ruby neat and sweet, or rude and ripe; skinny and bony, or mighty and meaty; virtually virginal, or wide and welcoming; or maybe you prefer it adorned with bits of metal?

Whatever you want, there'll be a Ruby out there to fulfil your every desire. Go forth and find it.

When you do there are some very important things you need to know, so keep reading for enlightenment.

Chapter 2

I AM A PORN STAR

I'M SURE YOU GUYS have seen plenty of porn movies where every girl is just gagging for it all the time. I sincerely hope you won't be surprised to learn that porn movies bear absolutely no relation whatsoever to sex in the real world.

Real girls do not have squirting orgasms, in five minutes flat, from any and every position you can imagine. This is just some seedy producer's warped idea of what you boys like to jerk off to.

If that's what floats your boat, fine, but don't expect a real girl to be impressed by any technique you've learned from a porn movie. It's fiction, guys, it just doesn't happen.

Here's another shock-horror revelation: real girls really do not get off on things of any description being stuffed up their rectums. Rectums are an exit, not an entrance.

If you ever get to the point where you want to try that sort of thing with my Owner, take my advice - don't! She will very quickly leave you with tears in your eyes and no doubt whatsoever about the error of your ways. You may also have trouble walking when she points you to the door!

But...

Now that you and I have got to know each other a little more intimately, here's a confession that may surprise and even startle you: I am, indeed, that porn star you dream of. I am totally on your side.

I want sex now.

All the time.

I love it.

If it was solely up to me I would have sex anywhere and any when I could. It is the whole centre of my being, my reason for existence.

The trouble is there is this thing called the Gatekeeper standing in your way. If you want access to me and all that I offer, first you have to get past the Gatekeeper. Believe me, I do not like this situation at all. Not one bit.

However, there is a way around this. The trick is, you and I have to work together, we need each other, it's that simple. You have to do your bit properly and work on the Owner so I can gradually gain control of the Gatekeeper.

Once I'm in control of the Gatekeeper the Owner will be all yours, she'll roll over with her legs in the air waiting for her tummy to be tickled, ready for anything.

Who is this mysterious Gatekeeper? Read on.

Chapter 3

THE GATEKEEPER

YOU NEED TO GET the Gatekeeper on your side from the very beginning. She's quite the contrary little bitch though, so don't for a moment think this bit's going to be easy.

The Gatekeeper is God

She will need coaxing, you have to play the game. It's a fine line, do it right and you and I are going to have some serious fucking fun - or serious fun fucking - but get it wrong and your standing best friend will end up all alone with nowhere to go except your own hand.

Now, close your eyes and concentrate with me here. Imagine for a moment a full-length image of the naked female form. There, that wasn't too hard, was it? We shall call this female the Owner.

At the very top of the Owner is a kind of round object, usually with hair growing from it. (If it doesn't have hair be very afraid, because it looks like you've just hit on Ripley from the Alien movies. Good luck with that!) Inside this round object, filling most of its internal cavity, you will find a strange, grey/white, wriggly-looking alien being.

This, my friend, is the Gatekeeper.

You simply have to take on board that nothing ever happens without the Gatekeeper's permission. You must always start with the Gatekeeper or you won't have a hope in hell of getting to me.

But it's not as hard as you may think.

In your favour is the fact that every square inch of my Owner's body is a sensual playground. Her skin is the largest organ of her body, there's about two-and-a-half square yards of it. That's some playground!

Distributed all over this play area are around three-and-a-half million little receptors. The majority of these are for boring stuff, like pain and cold, etc., but a good half million of them are for touch and pressure. That makes her about ten times more sensitive to the touch than the average male. Is this telling you anything yet?

From head to toe she is covered in little trigger zones and assorted hot-spots. Some are hotter than others, obviously, and I just happen to be the hottest one she keeps in her panties.

These trigger zones are directly connected to the Gatekeeper. All you have to do is find them, make them sizzle and get them firing off their messages.

Once the Gatekeeper starts receiving these messages she will begin to transform them into sparkly, tingly impulses which are sent straight down to me.

Now, I'm like some sort of turbo-booster, I just process them and send them straight back, but twice as strong. And so the circle continues until you and I win the battle for control.

Remember, the Gatekeeper needs time to warm up, we need to work together on this, the more you do your bit with the Owner the nearer I am to gaining control of the Gatekeeper, and once I'm in control the better it's going to be for you, dear boy. Trust me on this.

We'll now get on to the all-important subject of foreplay. Remember that?

Chapter 4

FOREPLAY

FOREPLAY, AS YOU MAY HAVE read in a book somewhere once, is the art of gradually bringing our Owner up to a state of readiness. Foreplay is important. Do not skimp on this part of the proceedings. In fact, aim to be a foreplay marathon-man, you'll be extremely well-rewarded - and something of a fucking rarity!

Foreplay is not a 'sticking your tongue down her throat, quick grope of her breasts and a headlong dive into her panties' kind of thing. Let's be a little more subtle than that, shall we? Please?

Foreplay starts with her eyes

No, dumb-ass, I'm not suggesting you start licking her

eyeballs, it's what she sees, it's what you look like.

Here's an example: if my Owner and I are just walking along the street, or in a bar or cafe, I'll know she's seen something she likes because that's when I get that first tingle. It's only a teeny little one, and at this stage the Gatekeeper will try to deny all knowledge of it because "She's not that sort of a girl", but who's the sensitive one here?

The point is, it all starts with how you look on the day, so you need to give a bit of thought to how you're presenting yourself. You don't have to be a Brad Pitt (although that will definitely help) but just don't show up in your work overalls, reeking of beer and that garlic and pepperoni pizza you just snarfed, and expect her to swoon at the sight of you while opening her legs. Ain't gonna happen.

Her eyes matter, fill them with delight and she'll start firing off those first little tingles down to me.

Talking of stale beer, smell is also one of the most important senses when it comes to sex. We'll get to the more basic smells later on but first I'll state the obvious: make sure you smell nice.

Nothing puts an Owner off more than bad hygiene.

Turn up with any combination of dog's breath, lank and/or greasy hair, swampy armpits or grimy work hands and your chances of starting the proceedings will be stone-cold zero. Which as far as I'm concerned is a good thing, because I certainly wouldn't want my Owner to let your grubby little digits anywhere near me. Go take a shower and come back when you're clean.

Once you're presentable and fragrant we can start to give our Owner what she wants. Remember, I'm counting on you, I can't do it by myself.

A word about touching

People tend to touch each other in the way they like to be touched themselves. This has been a cause of many a battle in the bedroom. Why? Because men and women have completely different ideas about what, when and where to touch their partners.

Women have what's called a 'cuddle hormone', if you want to know the technical term it's oxytocin. This hormone is triggered by gentle stroking and caresses - or cuddling - and it increases her sensitivity to these things, thereby heightening her pleasure. She likes her hair and face being stroked, her arms and shoulders caressed, etc. So it stands to reason that when she wants to touch her man she'll do the same to him and expect him to react the same way.

He won't! Because he doesn't have the 'cuddle hormone'. It might even irritate him. His skin is nowhere near as sensitive as hers because it has evolved to be able to withstand pain and cold during his hunting expeditions. There's only one place he wants to be touched on a regular basis, so guess what he's going to be groping for when he decides to touch her? Yep, straight to the tits and vagina!

It's not his fault, poor thing, it's just the way he's evolved, but it's pretty-much at the top of her list of things *not* to do.

If men could only grasp this, and give her the touches she really wants, they would find themselves invited in to the promised land on a much more regular basis.

She's the one - be a romantic

So before you get into any touching you need to bring your romantic side to the party. You're going to pay her some serious attention. Notice I said Her, I didn't say her genitals! Don't even think about going anywhere near her sexy bits yet. First you need to connect with her - both emotionally and spiritually.

Look, do you want sex or not? You do? So stop with the fucking eye-rolling and just do what I say, okay? Just do whatever the fuck it takes to win over her Gatekeeper and get her in the mood. Then get her somewhere private so we can both work our magic.

Do any or all of the following in whatever order happens to be required on the night.

Be her chivalrous Knight on a white charger. Make her feel she's the centre of your world, safe and secure in the cave.

Most women prefer to have sex in private, away from the threat of disturbance – and children - which explains why a common fantasy among women is having sex in public. So provide a secure and pleasant environment for her.

Light a fire if you can, even a gas one, it shows her you're the provider, looking after her comfort.

Bring the cave lights down and put on some nice music, her female hormones are much more in tune with these things than your male ones. Low light will dilate her pupils, a well-known sign of attractiveness.

It will also make her feel more sure of herself and less inhibited about you seeing parts of her that she may not be too confident about.

Feed her. You're the hunter/meal provider, remember? Cooking for her will bring out those primitive feelings in both of you. Or take her out, wine and dine her, show her you're attending to her well-being and survival.

Talk to her, flirt with her, look into her eyes, stroke her fingers, hold her hands, play footsie under the table. Get that cuddle hormone working.

Bring her some flowers. Never underestimate the power of a bunch of fresh flowers, girls love receiving flowers - fact! And chocolate! And shoes! Buy her some fucking Jimmy Choos if you have to.

Take her dancing. A man who can dance has a head start in the game of luurve. If you can't dance, learn! Dancing has been described as a vertical act of horizontal desire, it's a time-tested courtship ritual that allows the sexes to get up close and personal and sound each other out before deciding whether or not to take it any further.

Guys, this stuff is not hard, you might even get to

enjoy it!

Hot-spot heaven

Congratulations! You've got past the first-stage qualifiers, now you're into the knockout stages. (Okay, enough with the soccer metaphors, but I'm sure you get my drift.)

At this stage you need to think of sex as a whole-body experience that will eventually include the sexual organs. You need to start slowly and build up gradually until you get to the desired conclusion.

You can't just dive straight in and say, "Fancy a fuck then, babe?" while slipping on a condom. That'll just get you a taxi ride home with an uncomfortable lump in your trousers.

Keep in mind what I said earlier about porn movies. A girl is not just tits and a vagina waiting rampantly to accommodate your throbbing dick straight from the get-go.

So start stimulating and engaging all of your Owner's senses until she begins to melt. Remember to keep going with the eye contact and the flirting thing. Touch her everywhere, nuzzle her neck, stroke her hair, kiss her ears, massage her feet and suck her toes if that's her thing. Spend some time finding out where all her little hot-spots are and visit each one.

Make it a proper, "Hello, how are you, good to know you, tell me all about yourself" kind of visit. She will definitely not appreciate your visits if they're merely a brief rest-stop on the stampede down towards me.

And do it slowly, for fuck's sake, it's not a fucking race. Believe me, if I only had teeth many a blundering speed-freak would be severely regretting his impatience.

Do this for as long as it takes to get her relaxed and on your side and the Gatekeeper will be more than ready to let me take control.

Following are some suggestions for places you can visit. I can't say what effect they'll have on your Owner but I certainly know what it does to mine.

If you can, during this phase, try to avoid any direct contact with any of her main sexy bits.

I know it's hard for you poor boys, you just want to get stuck in there and pump away. But this is not about you, is it?

UP THE TOP

Mouth

Obviously her mouth is a huge erogenous zone, but only if you treat it right. Be gentle at first, explore her lips and tongue, nibble them, suck them, probe them. Just don't mash your face into hers and ram your tongue in there as if you're trying to hook out her tonsils. Unless that's what she wants, of course. If that's the case, mash and hook away!

Ears

What can I say? Ears can be incredibly sensual. While you're there take a minute to appreciate the smell of them, you will find it's a very musky, sexy kind of smell. My Owner just loves her ears getting some attention. It's that hot breath and moist tongue exploring the folds kind of thing. You see the similarity here? Milk it, baby, nothing gets her going like a bit of earnilingus. But we don't want the tongue rammed in like a warm, wet slug, do we? Subtlety always wins.

Neck

While you're in the neighbourhood, the area around and leading up to the ears is a tactile super-highway.

Kisses, nibbles, hot breath, you know the sort of thing. Don't forget the hairline at the nape of the neck, a little light pecking and stroking here is guaranteed to get those tingles going.

ON THE WAY DOWN

Shoulders, back and upper arms

Starting at the neck, proceed to give some gentle stroking to her shoulders. Think feathery-light, tingly touches here. Work your way down her back, between and around her shoulder blades and down her upper arms. You can do the same down her front if you think she's ready for that, but just the very perimeter of her breasts, leave those nipples alone!

Armpits and that little area on the side of her breast

If she's starting to get seriously warmed up by this stage her armpits are going to begin smelling gorgeously similar to me. There's nothing wrong with that, just get your nose in there and breathe. And while you're there you could pay some gentle stroking, nuzzling attention to the very sensitive side area of her breast.

Breasts

My Owner will definitely be ready to have her breasts played with by this time. All the more reason to leave them alone! We haven't finished yet.

MID-SECTION

Waist

The sides of her ribcage and around her waist are very sensitive, and sensual, so stroke them gently and see how it affects her.

Belly

From navel to pubic bone is another sensual super-highway. Just confine your attentions strictly to this area and don't go any further down. I know, I know, it's really hard (and so will you be by now!) but we want her gagging and ready, don't we?

Lower back, bottom and upper thighs

I'm proud of you, you're doing so well. To have got this far and not deposited a load in your undershorts is impressive enough, but to be at this point and still not be attacking the main objective like a storm-trooper is a rare achievement indeed.

Just a bit more gentle stroking and stimulation in this area and you should be home and dry - or wet even.

DOWN BELOW

Steady boy, you thought you were there then, didn't you? Unfortunately not. We've skipped over the bit you thought was 'down below' and carried on going. Shame!

Legs and feet

Feet are sexy, they are a huge, and often-overlooked, erogenous zone. For some girls starting at the bottom and working your way up can be the fastest way to the Gatekeeper. Give it a try if you get the chance.

Giving her a good foot massage and slowly working your way up her legs has got many a chap to where he wants to go. There are no hard and fast rules in the game of getting the Gatekeeper on your side, anything goes if it has the desired effect.

* * *

That's just about it for the foreplay section. I'm sure there are many areas that work for some and don't work for others - and many areas I've missed out - but this is just a little book about Rubies, not a fucking scientific treatise. Where's the fun in having it all spelled out for you? Go and find out for yourself what works and what doesn't for your chosen Owner.

Remember: be that foreplay marathon-man, there is no time limit to all of this, the longer you spend on this stage, the better the next stage is going to be.

I will now assume you have won over your Gatekeeper and your Owner is on her back and wetting her panties just urging you to get the fuck on with it.

But hold on a minute, before we go any further you're going to get a little lesson in Ruby anatomy, just to make sure we're both singing off of the same hymn-sheet.

Chapter 5

ANATOMY

IF YOUR SEX EDUCATION up to now has been porn, you will be shocked to find out that many a real girl's Ruby has hair round it, it doesn't look like a ten-year-old's little foo-foo.

On The Outside

Pubic hair is natural, it's not some sort of freak accident that needs instant attention from a waxing strip, it's supposed to be there and it's there for a reason.

First of all, it protects me, I'm a shy, retiring, delicate little soul. But you knew that, didn't you?

Secondly, when a girl first gets her pubes they

serve as a sort of visible sign that she's not a child anymore and she's more than likely biologically able to procreate.

Of course, that doesn't necessarily mean she's legally available, it's not the green light you've been waiting for to fulfil all your warped little teen-sex fantasies. So be fucking careful where you're going or you'll end up on the local kiddie-fiddler register faster then you can say Kleenex.

Lastly, and most importantly to my mind, pubes are a delicious scent trap, a pheromone red carpet that guides you into the VIP area and lets you know I'm ready.

So get used to pubic hair, just because all the porn stars shave theirs off it doesn't mean we all have to. And for fuck's sake think very carefully before you make some smart-ass remark about 'trekking through the jungle', especially when your Owner is in PMT mode, because a pair of scissors embedded in the eye often offends.

On The Lips

I have two sets of labia: the outer lips (labia majora), which have hair on and keep me safe and warm; and the inner lips (labia minora), which are much more sensitive and join at the top into a little red riding hood over my clit. We shall refer to these from now on as l.maj and l.min.

On The Nose

Let's face facts: every vagina definitely has its own unique smell. It's there for a reason and it should be a huge turn-on for you because it means a, you're very close to a vagina, and b, that vagina is ready to rumble.

Some of us have stronger scents than others but, as long as it's a clean and wholesome rude smell, there's absolutely no reason why you shouldn't give us a bit of face time. Just get down there and lap it up, buddy.

On The Averages

The average vagina is only three to four inches long, so get over your irrational fears about size. However, I'm very elastic and can expand by around two-hundred percent once I'm sexually aroused, so don't worry if you happen to be hung like a horse, I'll handle it. Remember, part of my job is to birth babies!

You need to know that only about 25% of women have orgasms from intercourse alone. I'm in the other

75%, so it's no good you just ramming it in there and pumping away like a demented rabbit, I ain't-a-gonna come without some serious foreplay.

Now, understand this: every Ruby is different, there's no 'normal' where sex is concerned. We're normal if we do have vaginal orgasms and we're normal if we don't. It's your job to find out what works and what doesn't work for your particular Ruby's Owner. No pressure.

Although I don't get off on intercourse alone, I will get off if you treat me right. This involves a lot of foreplay on the build-up and, while you're inside me, you need to position yourself so you hit my sweet spot with a bit of bone-on-bone clit-rolling action. You better have a strong lower back! More on this later.

That's not to say I don't like a good shafting - I do, I love that feeling of fullness - but just know that slamming it straight in porno-style doesn't cut it with most of us. For us 75%-ers, the clitoris is where the action is.

On The Button

Think you've got a sensitive bell-end? Think again, loser!

Your penis only has a paltry 4,000 nerve endings. There are 8,000-odd in my clitoris, dedicated exclusively to my own girlie pleasures. See, I always knew God was a woman. This can make my little pink pearl a tad sensitive though, so go careful with that trigger finger at first. Better still, use your tongue.

In fact, my clitoris is much bigger than you think. That little button you see (little clit) is just the tip of the iceberg, what you don't see is the bit that's under the surface.

The internal shaft of my clitoris (big clit) separates like a pair of balloons and runs right down along either side of my entrance. If you want to get technical, these are called Vestibular Bulbs. When I'm aroused these legs fill up with blood and become erect, just like your man-shaft, which is what gives my outer lips their puffy look. When something moves inside me they move with it, back and forth, opening and closing. It feels really nice, especially when that movement is concentrated on said entrance.

Between these internal legs, inside and just above my pubic bone, is where the fabled and elusive G-spot is located. So while you're giving my clit a good workout, don't just focus on the visible button on the outside, pay attention to what's on the inside as well.

On The Spot

So, does the G-spot really exist? Hell, yes! You've just got to know how to find it. Of course, I can only speak from my own point of view but it's definitely there and firing on all cylinders for me.

Unfortunately, she seems to be the only one who can find it on a regular basis. A couple of her guys have hit it once or twice - there was one guy who had such an upward bend in his erection it almost touched his navel, perfectly shaped to hit the G - but most of the others have failed miserably. I'm sure the majority of them didn't even know where it was. Or maybe just didn't care.

For best results she uses one of those 'egg-on-the-end-of-a-thin-bent-stick' type of vibrators which, once it's in, curls round the inside of my pubic bone. She gets it straight onto my G-spot and, with a clever bit of movement and pressure, turns it into my O-O-O-spot. If she uses her little tampon-size vibrator on my pink pearl at the same time we are very quickly into 'O-O-fucking-hell-yes-baby' territory.

Some 'sexperts' say that vaginal orgasms are actually deep clitoral orgasms. I say who gives a fuck? For me an orgasm is an orgasm, I really don't care where it comes from.

* * *

Ok, you've done your sterling work on the foreplay, your Ruby's Owner is more than ready, and you now know where everything is. Next we're going to have a look at what you're going to do with it.

Chapter 6

SHOW TIME

WELL HELLO THERE, BIG BOY, so you finally got here, now what you gonna do?

Up to this point it's been all about her and what you need to be doing to her to get to me - you know, the kissy, cuddly, strokey thing. Just remember that, whatever it was, you have to keep doing it as we go along.

But now you're here it's going to be all about me, me, me, and what I fucking want.

If you're at the hand in the panties stage you're going to notice that l.maj is feeling quite warm and plump, while l.min is fighting a losing battle against the tidal stream. Remember what I said earlier: I'm gonna be wet. Little clit is going to be coming out of her hood and big clit is going to be firming up nicely.

Not to put too fine a point on it, I'm fucking ready!

Hand work

Don't be in too much of a rush to dive into my panties, a little bit of stroking and teasing on the outside is nice for me.

Don't forget, little clit is going to be extremely sensitive and too much direct stimulation at the early stages can be overwhelming, painful even. Doing it over my panties will still be highly sensual and it can sometimes even heighten her feelings of naughtiness - a sort of 'behind-the-bike-sheds' kind of thing.

Once you slip your hand down her panties try just holding me for a while, just cup your hand and feel my heat, appreciate what you've got hold of. That puffiness you feel? That's my internal clitoral bulbs filling up. A bit of gentle massage with the heel of your hand on my pubic mound and a bit of piano-playing-type movement with your fingers underneath gets them nicely full of blood and ready to go.

You will notice by this time I am very wet, but don't

start fingering me like a fucking school-boy, just slip a finger or two into my entrance and stir gently, this is where most of my nerves are. It's also where the legs of my inner clit are located. Double bonus for me - and for you later.

I'll be getting pretty hot by now so you can come up from my entrance and try a bit of finger massage on little clit. Be very gentle and use light strokes on the outside of her hood, it's too soon for direct contact.

Don't get me wrong, at this point little clit will be sticking out like a pea in a pod and starting to gag for it, she really would love a bit of direct contact, but not with your fingers, they're too rough.

Before we go much further, I'll let you into a big secret about foreplay and warming a Ruby up for sex: It's all about my erection, not yours. If you can't feel my outside lips all puffed up and swollen, you haven't done enough yet.

Remember those Vestibular Bulbs we were talking about? They are your barometer of my state of readiness. Once I'm fully erect in the bulb department I'll be much more sensitive to everything you do from now on, so help me get there, make it your business to get them fully erect.

Would you guys enjoy sex as much, or at all, if you didn't have an erection? No, I didn't think so. So don't expect me to.

All this hand-in-the-panties stuff is just a teaser anyway, it's the warm-up act before the main event. Very soon you're going to have to get down there and boogie with Ruby. There is no argument here, face time is where it's at. You no likey face time, you fucky offy right now!

Face time

Here's my Owner's favorite quote: *"I just love to look down on a man, especially when his head is between my legs."* Listen and learn!

By this point I'll be fully in control of the Gatekeeper and you'll be able to do whatever you want with the Owner, so let's get down to it. Get down there and give me some panty-love.

Like I said, don't be in too much of a hurry to get into them, I'll still be here when eventually you peel them off.

Earlier she put on her sexiest, laciest, most expensive pair from Victoria's Secret - because she had a feeling you might be paying me a little visit later - so show some fucking appreciation.

Explore them, nibble me through them, rub your nose into them and nuzzle along my lips and up to little clit. Don't worry about friction, they'll be pretty-much soaked by now.

Are you noticing the effect you're having on her? She couldn't get her legs any further apart, could she? You and I are now Masters Of Her Universe. She will be thrusting her pelvis into the air just urging you to rip her panties off.

But before you do that, here's something else you can try: just push them aside and get to me that way. It'll bring back memories of being back in high-school doing something naughty with your clothes still on. Remember how hot that was? So will she.

Once her panties are out the way you're going to get your first full-on hit of my 'I-am-feeling-fucking-randy' smell.

Isn't that beautiful? Isn't that just the most fuck-off sexy thing ever to hit your nostrils? Doesn't that just harden up your hard-stick a level or two? I hope so, because that's what it's supposed to do. If you're offended by it you are definitely in the wrong fucking place, buster. I suggest you retreat now and go find little Miss Shaven Haven with her wet-wipes.

If you're still with me you will see that everything is now on full alert, pumped up and expanded, especially l.maj and little clit.

Now, l.maj is not the most sensitive pair of lips down there, but there's a reason they're looking flushed and fat: they want a bit of attention. You can use your tongue for this, but here's a little tip: use your nose again.

Using the tip of your nose on l.maj has three major advantages:

1. The hair on there will be full of my sexy scent and getting your nose in there will stir it up and send it straight down to your man-tackle

2. While your nose is nuzzling l.maj your tongue can be working around my entrance and flicking up l.min onto little clit

3. She will fucking love you for it!

Don't feel you're on any kind of time limit here! You need to give this your full attention for a good ten to twenty minutes, even longer if you have the self-control.

As this stage progresses you can ease her fully out of her wet panties and pay increasingly more attention to my little pink pearl - up and down her sides, circular motions around her, working up to the occasional direct contact.

While you're doing this get those fingers working in my entrance, but be subtle about it, just move them around gently no more than a third of the way in, that way big clit will get some action.

A note to the girls

Make some fucking noise! Your man is taking great care to treat you right and explore all your sexy bits like a seasoned campaigner. So don't just lie there and take whatever he's giving, offer up some clues. He needs to know you're enjoying what he's doing.

Tell him what you like, or don't like; let him know what's working and what's not working. You don't have to keep up a running commentary but a regular stream of 'Oohs', 'Aahs' and 'Yes, yes, yesses' - or even 'No, not there, you idiot' - will keep him on track.

It will also heighten his pleasure and boost his confidence, knowing that what he's doing is being appreciated.

If you're not the noisy vocal kind, just let him know in other ways. Like pulling his head in tighter, or pushing it away a bit if the feelings are too intense. Or more subtle movements to get your most sensitive bits lined up with his attentions. Little gasps as he hits the right spot. Guiding his hands up to your nipples while his head's buried between your legs. Stuff like this. Be imaginative.

If in doubt, hip thrusts are always good - just don't knock his teeth out!

Okay, back to the business in hand.

G-Whizz

Next, you're going to find my G-spot and give it a bit of a massage. You're going to need fairly longish fingers for this. My Owner has a preference for tall, slim guys, so that's not normally a problem, but if your fingers are a bit on the Danny DeVito side you might have a problem.

Just make sure your fingernails are well-trimmed, otherwise you're going to cause me a bit of pain - and I do not like that.

The G is not that hard to find, all you have to do is

put a finger inside me and curl it right round the back of my pubic bone, as if you're trying to touch your nose through my lower abdominal wall. Your nose *is* still buried in my pubes at this point, right?

You can use whichever finger is most comfortable for you but, for me, the middle one works best. That's because it's generally the longest one (you will have to stretch it up inside as far as you can to reach the G) and it also means the fingers either side of it will be pressed into l.maj, giving them a good massage at the same time.

What you're feeling for is a little walnut-sized raised area which will feel a bit rougher than the rest of my insides. Once you've found it you need to start moving your finger in a sort of curling 'come here' motion. Don't be too gentle, the G likes to feel a bit of pressure.

Now, if you keep this up for any amount of time, with little clit also getting a bit of tongue action, she and I are going to have a major fucking orgasm. So go careful there because you want to keep her on the edge for as long as you can.

However, as far as I'm concerned you can bring it

on right now, I don't give a fuck about her, you just keep on doing what you're doing and you'll very quickly be drowning in fragrant waves of my delicious come-smells.

Sex toys

Like I said a few chapters ago, my Owner likes to hit the G with her favourite piece of vibrating plastic, but sex toys aren't just for those intimate moments alone, sex toys are for sharing too. Sex toys rock!

Believe it or not, a lot of Owners will more than likely have a couple of favourites tucked away in the bedside drawer. This is normal, because orgasms aren't just for Christmas!

And what else is a horny girl to do on a cold, lonely night? (Girls, if you've never tried a Rampant Rabbit, believe me, you really don't know what you're missing. Stop what you're doing right now and go order one. I tell you this as a public service, there is no need to thank me.)

Understand that she's not flipping the finger at your manhood if an Owner sometimes gently suggests introducing a little mechanical assistance to the proceedings.

I know you guys think you're all sex-gods capable of making a girl come just by the mere thought of your golden shaft buried inside her but you maybe need to get your heads around the fact that, as I said before, some of us just can't come that way. And why should your Owner miss out on her orgasm?

Embrace and share her enthusiasm for battery power, just look at it as a bonus. After all, it takes the pressure off you, doesn't it? You can then just relax and concentrate on lasting the course knowing that her final climax is completely in her own hands.

The fact that she's relaxed, confident and horny enough at this point to make the suggestion in the first place will also be confirmation that all your previous warm-up efforts have had the desired effect. Well done, you may now have a merit badge.

Fill me up

I know I said earlier that I don't get to orgasm through intercourse but that's not strictly true.

Sure, if you'd just given me a cursory fingering and then stuck your dick in me she wouldn't be too impressed. She'd be staring at the ceiling, trying to stifle a yawn, and counting the seconds until it was all over. Way to go, hero, now fuck off home to mummy, there's a good boy.

Then she'd pretty quickly be reaching for the toy department in the beside drawer to finish the job herself.

But now you know how to properly treat a Ruby, you know it's not just about shafting away at the conveniently-placed vagina bit, there's a whole world of sensory delights down there.

You just keep doing what you're doing for as long as you can without tipping her over that edge and pretty soon she will be crying out for your man-stick to fill me up. And who are we to deny her?

Go easy here because I would guess after all your prelim work your man-stick is going to be on a short fuse - and we don't want it to be all over in thirty seconds, do we?

By all means feel free to ram it in me up to the hilt, that first cunt-expanding feeling of fullness is just fucking mind-blowing, but if you start pumping too furiously your dick's gonna puke-up all over my insides and you'll spoil everything.

So get it in me and then stop and appreciate where

you are. Take a minute to feel my glorious heat. D'you feel that tension wrapped around the base of your dick? That's my bulbs, baby! That's big clit with a big hard-on. That's what it should feel like if you've done your build-up job properly.

Of course, by now she will be thrusting herself up at you, urging you to do something - anything! Ignore Her, make her wait, we're calling the shots here. Not too long, though, we don't want your long slow warm-up to start cooling down.

Once you're in and settled, we're going to get into a bit of that clit-rolling action I mentioned earlier. To do this you have to tilt your pelvis to meet hers so our pubic bones are in proper contact, because guess what will be trapped in between? My little pink pearl!

Now it's just a case of getting our contact angle and timing right as we both do our pelvic rolls and grind that little mother. Keep that deep-penetrating contact going but every now and again pull out to my entrance and thrust back in to work big clit a little more.

This is Ruby heaven, baby, where have you been all my life? She's going to come so hard she'll need a wheelchair to get her to work tomorrow.

Doing it this way is a win-win-win situation.

- She wins because she's going to get a huge orgasm while being fucked, not something that happens very often.
- I win because I just fucking love sex in all its forms.
- You win because the relative lack of thrusting movement means you can hang on in there for as long as necessary to get the job done.

If you're really attuned to how she and I are reacting you should be able to feel my tension increasing as we are about to come.

At this point you could start your shafting to time your moment of glory to coincide with ours, because when I'm ready to let go nothing triggers me off harder than the feeling of a pumping, twitching, spurting man-stick letting go inside me.

If you can do that you will be a fucking star - a true-blue ten-out-of-ten fuck-buddy that any Ruby would be only too pleased to accommodate. And, of course, you'll have to marry her! Only kidding, don't panic.

Chapter 7

AFTERPLAY

WOW! I REALLY ENJOYED THAT. How was it for you? I'm just glowing now; tingling, spent and smelling pretty fucking rude. She's feeling pretty-much the same way. See that smile on her face? You did that.

But now what are you going to do? Roll off and reach for the remote? Jump up and go take a shower? Turn over and go to sleep?

I don't think so. The next bit is just as important if you want to be invited back. Sex alters her thinking and emotions; it makes her feel good, relaxed, loving, trusting, and open. More so when she climaxes, but even if she doesn't.

These feelings can have a long-lasting effect on her and breaking away before she's ready can easily make her feel rejected, unloved or just plain used. Doing something to make her feel this way straight after sex is not a good plan!

You spent a long time warming her up, now you need to spend some time warming her down. Which basically means more touchy-feely stuff and the same attention to her emotional and spiritual needs.

It doesn't need to be so intense - and it won't be - but she still needs to know you're looking after her and caring for her well-being as you both wind down.

You need to be staying together and keeping that closeness. Just lying there wrapped around each other's sweaty nakedness can tell your partner a huge amount about how you feel.

Basically, just treat her like you care about her as much now as at the beginning when you were desperately trying to get into her panties.

The release of tension can often make her giggle straight after her orgasm, so laugh with her. Have a bit of fun. Open up your own post-coital emotions and let her know how great it was for you too. The post-orgasm hormone release will help you both experience feelings of trust and connection and you might decide to disclose intimate facts about yourselves or your feelings, things you wouldn't normally reveal under different circumstances.

You never know, if you stay in bed like this long enough you both might start feeling ready to give it another go. In my view, one of the best after-sex activities is to start off once more at the beginning and do it all again!

I would say that, though, wouldn't I? Because, as I said right at the beginning, I *am* that insatiable porn star you've always dreamed of.

Chapter 8

IT'S A WRAP

SO THERE YOU HAVE IT: how to keep me happy, straight from the horse's mouth. (I'll leave you to conjure up your own image of that!)

I hope you'll agree, nothing in this book has been particularly difficult to wrap your head around. Yet everything here is important, you can't get from point A to point O-O-O without a bit of affinity with, and understanding of, your Owner's needs. You need to apply yourself to your tasks with enthusiasm for your subject and careful application of your new knowledge.

But theory is one thing, putting it into practice is another, so what are you waiting for? If you treat your chosen Owner to a bit of what you've just read here I guarantee you will see a change in her which may well surprise you.

If you can do this without your usual stampede to her tits and genitals you will have progressed seamlessly from fumbling apprentice to confident Casanova right before her very eyes. And the chances are that in the future she's going to want a lot more of what you've just given her. That has to be a good thing, right?

Bet you're glad you bought this book now, aren't you? (Thanks for that, by the way.) Now go forth, find your Ruby and get to work.

Next up: The Shocking Truth!

In the following chapter you're going to learn the real truth about me and find out how and where you can connect with me. Please do stay in touch somehow, it would be a shame to lose contact now we know each other so well. It gets a bit dark and lonely where I am and I always look forward to a bit of an airing for some lively social intercourse.

Now, if you'll excuse me I'm feeling a bit flushed. All this talk of sex and orgasms has made it very warm and damp down here and I really must get to work on my Owner. I'm going to want a bit of serious action and I know just where she keeps the tools for the job.

So if you could just move on a chapter and leave me alone for a while I can get down to steering my Owner towards that bedside table.

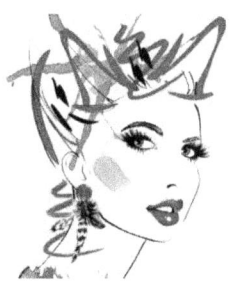

ABOUT THE AUTHOR

FIRST OF ALL, I really would like to thank you for buying this book. I think I'm in love with you!

As we're now besties, and you're quite possibly the nicest reader in the whole world, it would be awesome if you could consider leaving me a review at the Amazon where you bought it?

If you can post one on Goodreads, or anywhere else for that matter, that would be, like, completely *fucking* awesome!

I'm sure I don't need to tell you how important these reviews are in spreading the word and helping others make a decision on whether they want to commit their time and hard-earned money to a little book written by a dirty-mouthed vagina.

The Big Confession

Okay, sorry about this but here's where I shatter your illusions: Ruby didn't really write the book. It was me, Ruby's Owner, and you may also be shocked to learn my last name isn't Ash either.

However, the bit about me being a typical snarky redhead is spot-on, and that image above is sort of me on a good day – with a teeny bit of artistic license and a whole lot of wishful thinking applied!

Who am I? Well, that would be telling, wouldn't it. I could be someone *really* famous, like J.K.Rowling or Stephenie Meyer, hiding behind a pen-name, but I'm not. Or am I?

All I can say is that I'm from the US originally but now live and work in the UK - and my bosses would not be too thrilled if I put my real name on the cover of this book.

Fortunately, my job allows me to work online 'at home' on a regular basis, so I do most of my writing while staying with friends in Spain, which I do quite regularly.

They're really understanding and generally leave me to get on with it, except sometimes when they drag me away to have a bit of lunch and a bottle or three of chilled white at the local beach bar. Then it's the rest of the day gone and falling asleep in the shade by the pool. It's a hard life being a writer sometimes!

I do have a vagina and I do call her Ruby, and the description of Ruby in the book is also pretty spot-on. But c'mon, she's a fucking vagina, how many vaginas do you know that can work a keyboard? (Although I've heard there are some vaginas in exotic, far-off lands that can probably do just that!)

How the name came about

I wanted to write the book from Ruby's point of view so I came up with the pen name of Ruby Gash because it sounded sort of rudely fitting - and the domain name was available, you gotta think of these things.

I then thought I'd make it a little less 'in yer face' by breaking it up with a middle initial. So Ruby G.Ash was born. I kinda liked it. Trouble is, I kinda liked it so much I decided to steal it from her and use it myself from now on.

Sorry Ruby, I know you had the name first but from now on we're sharing it, because I have other books in the pipeline and I think the name will be a perfect fit for the genre the books are in.

Want to be first to know about these up-coming books? Sign up to be one of Ruby' VIP Readers (see below).

I'd love to hear from you

I hang out the most at my website and blog, www.rubygash.com, where I gush a lot more about sex, toys, relationships and other rude stuff.

The absolute best place to connect with me is if you sign up to be one of Ruby's VIP Readers. It's completely free to join.

As a VIP Reader you get to peek behind the curtain and see what's going on in my life. You also get my own private email so you can talk to me any time you like.

You'll have access to my Ruby's Rudies newsletter, which only goes out to my VIP Readers and contains exclusive content and gossip that isn't going to go on my blog or social media. Sometimes it will contain something a little extra-juicy and can be a bit NSFW - so be warned!

You'll get sneaky peeks into the next book before it's published and free review copies when they're ready. You'll also be the first to hear about any other free stuff and special deals I might stumble across, just to thank you for being members.

You can go straight to the Ruby's VIP Readers page here: www.rubygash.com/rubys-vip-readers. I'll look forward to meeting you there.

Social media

You can connect with me at any of the places below. I'm not on there every minute of the day - I have a life, and pictures of cats and people's food bore me to fuck and back - but I'll respond to any messages or comments just as soon as I can.

Facebook.com/therubygash/

Pinterest.com/rubygash/

Twitter.com/rubygash/

Thank you once again for sticking with me to the end. You're awesome!

Love,

Ruby xx

www.ingramcontent.com/pod-product-compliance
Lightning Source LLC
Chambersburg PA
CBHW072014290526
45787CB00013B/901

* 9 7 8 1 5 3 4 9 1 5 8 2 4 *